A.L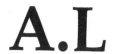

How to Transform
Your Cells and Yourself
from Disease to Wellness

A.L.I.V.E.

How to Transform
Your Cells and Yourself
from Disease to Wellness

By Dr. Stephanie J. Clark

ISBN: 978-0-9884471-6-5

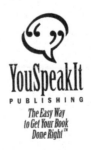

YouSpeakIt
P U B L I S H I N G
The Easy Way
to Get Your Book
Done Right™

www.YouSpeakItPublishing.com

Dedication

To all my former patients in Andalusia, Illinois; to patients who have participated in my ALIVE program; and to my family for all their love and support of my gifted ways.

Acknowledgments

I extend my deep gratitude to the following for helping me with this book:

Emit and Aspen, my two sons, who have changed me as a person to have a better understanding of gratitude.

Nathan, who consistently challenges my morals, standards, and values, and who has not only helped bring the ALIVE program to the next level with his Health and Life Coaching Guidance, but who pushed me to finish the print version of the program.

Dr. Timothy Gay, mentor and coach, for continued guidance during a new chapter of my life. Without your guidance, I would have struggled with balancing a career with motherhood. After introducing me to Michael Gerber, my wings were able to soar higher than ever before.

Michael Gerber. *The Dreaming Room* opened my eyes to imagined impossibilities of life. It allowed me to get outside myself and create the ALIVE program to profoundly help others get to a better place in their own lives.

Dr. Harry Wallace — mentor, friend, and colleague — the walking encyclopedia who guided my implementation of chiropractic care while at Palmer College of Chiropractic.

Toby, my best friend from childhood who has always been there. I still remember studying on your couch in college and you teasing me that I would become a doctor someday!

Stacy, Laura, and Mimi. Who could ask for better sisters?

Mom and Dad, for giving to so many people without expecting anything in return. For never giving up on yourselves, your children, and all the people you have both helped over the years. You are truly inspiring.

YouSpeakIt Publishing, who has provided the opportunity to complete my book seamlessly.

The Palmer Gang, all the Palmer College faculty and colleagues who were present while I attended school. It was an amazing experience.

The Camp Gang. All our healthy and unhealthy adventures help confirm the components of the ALIVE Program.

All the dis-eased, unhealthy, or healthy individuals who are looking for the next phase of health transformation. Enjoy the journey.

Contents

CHAPTER FOUR

CHAPTER FIVE

Introduction

As to methods, there may be a million and then some, but principles are few. The man who grasps principles can successfully select his own methods. The man who tries methods, ignoring principles, is sure to have trouble.

~ Ralph Waldo Emerson

ALIVE is a program for healing that I designed after years of observation of my patients, people with health challenges, and my own health challenges: a form of dyslexia, learning disabilities, slow cognitive function, food allergies and sensitivities, ovarian cysts, polycystic ovary syndrome (PCOS), and thyroid problems.

ALIVE is an acronym for the five categories that participants explore:

- Addictions
- Life
- Innate Intelligence
- Visions
- Emotions

Many people complain daily of ailments or personal drama.

It may be:

- Lack of money
- Job inadequacies

- Personal relationships
- A variety of health concerns

In the United States, the following ailments are all on the rise:

- Sleep apnea
- Anxiety
- Depression
- Headaches
- Vertigo
- Autoimmune diseases
- Autism
- Fibromyalgia
- Addictions
- Environmental allergies and sensitivities

Have you ever thought about the reason for your headache, disease, ache or pain, or why you are unhappy day in and day out?

Are you just treating the symptom, managing your disease — or are you correcting the problem?

Have you *become* your disease because a doctor informed you there was no alternate route of care?

When is enough enough?

How long are you willing to continue feeling miserable?

More than one patient has begun their care with me by stating they don't need my help: their disease is under control with medication or their blood labs are normal. Yet they are sitting in front of me in a state of *dis-ease* (a chiropractic term meaning lack of ease or harmony within the body). This is what the mainstream medical approach has trained us to understand and accept.

"Take this pill and your system will manage a disease."

What would happen if you did not take the pill?

Blood pressure and diabetes seem to be two of the more common conditions that receive a verbal response of ."management." By this I mean that these individuals typically make no lifestyle changes. They and their doctors manage their disease with medication. These patients are dependent on daily medical intervention.

Why do so many people accept this method of disease care that we call healthcare?

It is the easy way of not solving an underlying problem. It means you don't have to take responsibility for your own health or take action to gain a different result.

We learn about pill consumption from many sources:

- Healthcare providers
- Pharmaceutical companies
- The media
- Schools training healthcare professionals

Maybe we learn from a combination of all of them. The healthcare system has been tampered with to promote financial gains of others. What is not recognized is the cost of these gains. The loss is not felt by the pharmaceutical and insurance companies, but by the consumers — the patients who are seeking help.

The insurance companies are there for coverage in the medical model when you are diseased or injured. Preventative coverage is limited.

Have you ever gone to your doctor complaining of a symptom, and when all your blood labs were normal, you were sent home only to be called back three months later to be retested?

You are left still not feeling well; meanwhile, you become more and more dis-eased. Our cellular health and function are being compromised to the point of *apoptosis*, cellular death.

My own health challenges started in high school, after a car accident left me with a knee problem. It cost me the ability to play lacrosse that season, when I was at the peak of my career. I was referred to a physical therapist who gave me the tools to rehabilitate my knee back to playing status. I played the last game of the season. It was then that I realized I wanted to devote my career to helping people get their lives back like the physical therapist helped me get mine.

Over the years, I have come to understand that health is much more than rehabilitation. While I was in college studying physical therapy, movement therapy, and sports and exercise science, I was diagnosed with a cyst on my ovaries, and the recommended treatment was surgery to remove the ovaries.

I was barely nineteen years old.

My mom questioned the plan of action. She was concerned that I wouldn't be able to have children.

Before a decision was made, I ended up in the hospital with stomach spasms four times within the next six months. Fortunately for me, the ER doctor diagnosed me with food allergies that were causing my stomach problems. He also thought the cysts developing on my ovaries could be connected.

I was sent home with a bottle of liquid medicine that I was supposed to take every time my stomach spasmed. I finished half the bottle of medicine within eight hours, since my stomach was spasming every five minutes.

After not being able to function — not even being able to get off the couch — I realized I was going to have to take charge of my health. I had to find an alternate way to heal my stomach and my body. Mainstream medicine was not going to heal my cells.

I started changing my diet and my daily habits. I went to massage school. In massage school, I scored 98 percent on a neurological examination. My teacher, Dr. Robert Berube, was amazed and said no one had ever scored that high. He thought I should go to chiropractic school.

I was worried because I had battled with dyslexia all my life.

Despite my worries, I did go to chiropractic school. There, I learned another component of health in the neuroendocrine system: nerve function. The power of the nerve function in healing disease is not acknowledged enough.

Chiropractic is still not completely recognized for its value in making adjustments. I feel to this day that some of my dyslexia problems were due to food and nerve function, and after being under chiropractic care, my disabilities have changed. If I miss an adjustment, my disabilities will resurface.

After working with Michael Gerber in *The Dreaming Room*, I awakened to imagine the possibilities of the missing pieces I had observed over my years in practice — the missing pieces to health that, ironically, are organized mathematically.

I woke one night having found the missing pieces. I recognized that there is an organized cellular function. It has a mathematical universal component based on the number five. That was the beginning of the ALIVE program, which targets the multiple facets of organized matter.

Looking at the functionality of cells and matter and relating that to life forces, organizational expression and cellular interactions are mathematically expressed by the number five. There has to be balance in all five categories to maintain a healthy functioning cell.

Our healthcare system is great when people are in a measurably diseased state in which their cells are too sick to return to health. But we must change the trend toward disease and misery to a journey toward health and wellness. We have to learn to look at things differently. My hope is that by sharing the ALIVE program, we can educate people across the United States and across the world to be more proactive than reactive with their health.

Freedom lies in new neuronal connections throughout the body and brain. We are all born with the same amount of neurons in the brain, but it is the expression of the neurons that are affected by external and internal environmental stimulus.

For example, think about children learning to crawl. They may initially be able to lift their heads on their own, move an arm, then a leg, and eventually they'll be able to stand up and walk.

The developmental phase of crawling is designed to develop the myelin sheaths around the nerve. The myelin sheath is used to create *action potential* of a nerve. This is a chemical reaction that occurs to transmit and connect information along a nerve pathway.

Information can be about a:

- Thought
- Emotion
- Movement
- Function

The more you use a pathway, the more neurons will connect to that pathway.

Research has shown that over time, neurons will change pathways based on repetition. If you lose the myelin sheath around the nerve, you lose the ability to function.

[This is what happens to multiple sclerosis (MS) patients. After studying nerve function so extensively in chiropractic school, I have always thought that MS could be tied to pathogens, toxins, nutrition, gut health, or a combination of all components. For years, researchers have not been able to connect a specific cause. The newer research connects compromised gut health causing an increase in permeability in the gut lining. When this occurs, all of the above can be a combined cause.]

Repetitive neuron transmission changes over time. Consider the following two examples:

EXAMPLE NUMBER ONE

Have you had a thought that you could not get out of your head?

This often happens with thoughts that concern emotions.

One of our program participants as a little boy had been told by his father that he was stupid. That thought stayed with him, causing an increase in neuronal communication along that pathway. This affected his daily functions and actions as he grew older.

When he went to school, he would revert to the thought: *You are stupid.*

He was never able to complete a task or function because he always believed that one thought; he listened to that one neuronal pathway.

The repeated neuronal transmission became a debilitating emotional thought. He turned to drug and alcohol use to avoid dealing with this emotional pathway of failure. His own thoughts affected his success, but not his brain capacity.

The pathways of the brain have to be completed no matter what — information has to be routed. The brain does not know the difference between an emotion and a substance, as long as it takes the same pathway. This is why addictive behavior patterns occur. We can all accomplish greatness, but we get fixated on an emotion or point in time.

EXAMPLE NUMBER TWO:

When I was younger, my family hosted foster children.

Two girls came to live with us for a year. The older child had been sexually abused and her behaviors and interactions with her younger sister reflected that. She would act out the same patterns of abuse toward her sister.

My parents had to consistently redirect and reeducate the older sister that her behavior was unacceptable and not normal. Over time, she was able to break her behavior patterns, because the neuronal maps informed new neurons to change the actions. They were able to make a shift inside the brain.

This is why repetition is key to learning behaviors.

When antibiotics were discovered, we thought we had answered all our health concerns. So far, we have created more strands of bacteria. We have to go back to the earth for our healing properties and stop man from manipulating food, drugs, and chemicals around us. Human manipulation of products, goods, and services are coming at a cellular cost.

In your daily life, what affects your cellular function?

We are continually bombarded with stimuli, and usually, we don't realize what cellular functions are innately happening within our bodies. For instance, we don't even realize that our blood is pumping unless our blood pressure gets really high and puts increased stress on our heart. We don't usually think about cell function unless something goes wrong.

ALIVE is designed to set people free from unhealthy conditions and diseases. It targets different areas of external and internal environments to help rid disease, or challenges, within the cells.

- Some patients are looking for a specific resolution to an already-diagnosed condition.

- Other patients have a debilitating symptom that prevents them from even leaving their own house, but no test or prior doctor has found any abnormality.

- Some people are seeking support for their whole body and internal systems because they feel like the regular health model takes pieces and parts, and doesn't look at them as a whole.

The ALIVE program can potentially be used in all different medical facilities around the country. My vision is that I'm writing this for current patients, for those who feel as though they have no other avenues, and beyond the patients, to also make a change and impact in our disease care system that we call a healthcare system.

The book has five different chapters, and within each, five key components are specified that can impact your nervous system and the health and function of your cells. Though each chapter is separate, they all interconnect and interrelate.

When you read through the book, review each chapter and see how each one connects to another. It will help you to heal your system and make your cells more vibrant and less dis-eased over time. Reading this way will be very useful in changing your cellular function. It will help you become more aware of how you see the world and how your cells are receiving the world.

I'm hoping that as you read this, you can rethink what's going on in the universe and open your mind to alternative care, especially if mainstream, conventional medicine has not given you the results you were expecting.

My goal is to educate patients and their families so we can help ourselves and others get to a better place through daily function. As a nation, our internal health, organ function, and daily emotional stability are declining. We really need to educate people differently, or we're all going to be miserable. If people don't have the opportunity or resources to make a change, then they're not going to know how to do something different.

While reading the book:

- Take note of each category.
- Jot down how it applies to your life or others around you.
- Notice the implication of disease in your life.

As an example, let's say you have a really healthy diet,

but you still don't feel well. You can eat all the best foods, but that doesn't mean that your body is processing the food that you're taking into your system. It's important to look at each component — not only what you eat, but also how you are able or not able to digest — to see how they apply individually or in connection with each other.

Cell function can change even by subtle input that you may not notice, for instance:

- Fluctuation of voice
- Change in temperature
- Memory or past pattern that is emotionally significant

You may take them for granted and miss the opportunity to look at those little pieces. Those pieces can really impact your life and your health.

The goal of this book and my program is to help you recognize:

- How your body functions
- Why your body functions
- How the function of your cells can change

In my life, I've been fortunate to go through a process with healing my own body in different manners. Additionally, I've worked with patients, providing tools and new education strategies to get them to a better place. A lot of people strive their whole lives to find their purpose. Through a tragedy, I had the opportunity to find my purpose in life and help you find yours.

ALIVE helps you to:

- Identify missing pieces affecting your cellular function
- Start the repair process of cellular connection to external and internal stimulus
- Discover what parts of your life can improve

Try to find the good in every situation, good or bad. I found the good in the tragedy I lived through and feel very fortunate for that. I am able to help people get healthier and find their own way. There's not one way to do anything. I am grateful that I can wake up every day and work with people and have the passion to do it.

I hope reading this book creates a shift toward recovery and wellness in your own life, and helps you to put yourself in a better physical, mental, and spiritual state of mind.

CHAPTER ONE

Addictions

I want first to define *addiction* in reference to the ALIVE program.

The American Society of Addiction Medicine defines it the best:

> Addiction is a primary, chronic disease of brain reward, motivation, memory, and related circuitry. Dysfunction in these circuits leads to characteristic biological, psychological, social, and spiritual manifestations.

Addictions are prevalent in our society. They can be debilitating in even basic daily activities and skills, like getting dressed in the morning, eating, and thinking. If you live with addiction, your cellular and neuronal communication will be compromised.

Addictions come from the need for neurons to connect or from a reaction to the body's disconnection. Neuronal connections start in the womb and develop based on emotional connections with parents, siblings, and family members. When you were a child, you strategized to fit into your world based on how people interacted with you. Neuronal pathways and connections were formed and then carried through to your adult years.

Because you are bombarded with a lot of different stimulation in your environment, you may experience complications with your neuronal connections. These contribute to an increase in addictive behavior patterns.

Complications can arise in:

- Daily functions
- Personal relationships
- Mental coping skills

Children express behavior patterns in search of loving interactions. Childhood fears can stem from caregivers' reassurance to help soothe them. If as an infant or young child you did not receive love, neurological pathways may have developed with emotional trauma.

As you age, you look for other self-gratifying components to fulfill the love pathway you have been looking for since childhood. The brain does not know the difference between love and addiction. Both create the same neurological stimulation. If you do not feel loved or appreciated, you will seek the same feeling by way of an addiction.

One patient I worked with experienced the loss of a family member. They ended up moving to a different area, thinking that a new environment would make all of their problems go away. But they created the same problems in the new area, because they never dealt with the root cause of their problem. Until they deal with the death, they will continue to have the same problems.

You were born with genes that can express themselves in different ways. The genes can be affected by internal and external environmental stimulus. Addictions are external stimuli masking an internal emotion. Neuronal communication has the ability to receive and send information and can change over time. It's very important that we make and receive strong love impressions when we're younger, so that we're not as prone to addictive behaviors as we mature. Dopamine is one of the more important neurotransmitters that affects the brain-motivated reward system. Your body will try to produce dopamine in any way it can. The following five categories are the most common causes of dopamine release.

SEX

Sex addiction has increased with more exposure to pornography through TV and the Internet. You see more and more images that are going to change the neurological pathway of sexual interactions. In this circumstance, over time, your sexual arousal shifts from a feeling-type to a visual-type of arousal and interaction.

This means your normal level of arousal with feeling develops a need for visual stimulation, like pornography. There's a tipping point in the brain at which the neurotransmitters no longer function with the same pathways as they did when they were affected by touch. Eventually, in order for that neurological connection to occur, they can only transmit the information in the body through visual input. This is why, over time, the more you look at pornography, the more difficult it is to achieve arousal with your partner using touch.

This can present a lot of complications in a relationship. It can create communication problems. Because emotional and physical abuse cause a detachment between neurons, you will stay in protective survival mode in which you don't want to be touched or you have a heightened sex dive. The lack of closeness or forgetfulness of the past, a survival tactic of the brain, enhances sexual behavior patterns. Touch is more intimate and opens up exposure to being hurt.

The other partner may be experiencing thoughts like:

I'm not good enough.

My body's not good enough.

I'm not stimulating my partner.

The key to getting out of a sexual addiction is to develop a strategy for how to change that neurological communication back into the feeling realm instead of the visual realm. It involves loving the self, so you can be loved by another. That creates an additional emotional implication of how that can tie into the dis-eased state of the body that will be reviewed in Chapter Five: Emotions.

Changing sexual behavior patterns really comes down to the same biochemical process that occurs with any of the addictions that we talk about.

- You have a craving that your body is trying to satisfy.
- Your body's neurons have to make a proper connection for you to get a chemical shift.
- When your body doesn't make that connection, you feel that you need more.

The traditional approach to dealing with addiction has been by talking to the people who struggle with it. We tend to try to educate them and to show them different ways to do things, but we don't usually work with that biochemical pathway at the same time that we're trying to educate them about their external world. We don't address their internal world to try to shift their chemistry at the same time. That's where the value comes in if you want to really change an addictive behavior pattern, especially in the area of sexuality.

In my experience over the years, for the patients who had complicated relationships with sexual interactions, most of the cause was past childhood experiences that were not resolved. People unable to commit to or have monogamous relationships typically have unresolved emotional issues with someone or some experience from childhood.

GAMBLING

Gambling can be a very addictive behavior. Gambling is more of an outlet to relieve anxiety in the system then to stimulate the pleasure pathway. A gambling addiction can be very destructive for a family because it is harder to detect. Neurologically, the addiction to gambling occurs along the same pathway as drug addiction. Dopamine is released more with near misses than with wins.[1]

You have the visual stimulus of gambling in a facility that has slot machines. You visualize how to win money. In this situation, there is a reward system based on financial gain. If you are addicted to gambling, you are trying to solve your biochemical needs with money as your gain. The insula of the brain is affected more in gambling addicts.

Media constantly toss out new ways to spend money:

- The latest cell phone
- The newest computer
- The greatest tool for the job you need to do

The media puts a lot of pressure on you so that you'll feel as though you need to have these things. You might feel as though you need to make more money to be able to pay for these things too. You look for a quick fix, the easy way out.

1 L. Clark, Lawrence, A.J., Astley-Jones, F., Gray N. Gambling near-misses enhance motivation to gamble and recruit win-related brain circuitry. Neuron. 2009; 61(3):481-90.

You tell yourself: *I'll just gamble and I'll win a million dollars.*

We all know that that is not the way to earn money. You will probably end up losing more money in the long run. Then once you've lost that money, you keep going back for more, because now you don't have another money solution.

Trying to make easy money can be very debilitating. There's a certain amount of work that needs to be done to make a gain in life. Most people understand this, but those with a gambling addiction don't understand it completely or they don't have the coping skills to be able to figure out a different way.

Gambling shares many characteristics with other addicting activities:

- It changes your chemistry.
- You become more focused on visual stimulus.
- It stimulates the reward system.

Combine these attributes, and it's really hard to break out of the addiction. You must shift your focus on the tools and strategies to obtain a *new* reward system.

Look at the roots of the impulses.

Why are you in debt?

Why are you gambling?

Are you gambling for the high, or are you gambling for the financial success?

If you get help to figure out why you are gambling and what the reward is, then you can set up a different reward system that will follow the same chemical pathway. Once you set up that different reward system, then you can keep the proper stimulus that your body needs while you're educating yourself to make a shift in your life. Remember the change in behavior comes with the change to your brain chemistry.

That's the key: You need to provide a shift in the chemistry so you're still getting that good feeling. Returning to the addicting behavior is an attempt at regaining it.

SHOPPING

People are very unhappy with themselves and their situations. We are a society seeking instant gratification. We don't recognize that happiness comes from within and takes work. Shoppers are usually trying to fill an emotional void. If shopping is your addiction, you are trying to find yourself through your buying experience.

You may try to strategize about how to find happiness, so you:

- Buy a car
- Buy a chair
- Think a new rug is going to make you happy

Buying something will shift the chemistry to make you feel good at that moment, but how long is that new rug really going to satisfy you?

How long is that new car going to satisfy you?

You might still be miserable and unhappy, because you're not happy with yourself.

Take a look at how you feel about:

- How you cope with your partner
- Your satisfaction in your job
- Where you are living

Instead of feeling and experiencing the misery of your reality and why your system and your thought process feel that way, you try to find your identity and way through shopping. You are lost.

You are continually bombarded with marketing strategies to sell you the new clothes, the newest, latest, and greatest Fitbit, or other gadgets or status symbols you must have. I think TV commercials are now longer than the airtime for shows!

This widespread marketing tool creates a visual impact on your brain that says, "Come buy me, and then you'll feel better."

But actually, buying doesn't always make you feel better. Spending money just creates one more problem. Say for instance that you find you shouldn't have bought the new item. Maybe you can't afford it, or when you get it home it doesn't provide the same emotional satisfaction you felt at the time of purchase. So then that creates another emotion and problem within your brain-reward system. That then causes you to go shop or buy again. You think that you need the newest stuff because it will provide a happier life for you.

Shopping tends to be a compulsive behavior.

You go out looking for new socks.

You come home with:

- New socks
- A pair of shoes
- A new purse
- A new hat

And that's all because of the stimuli around you.

It's important to ask yourself:

Where was the shift in my life that created this need?

What changed that didn't provide something for my brain-reward system?

What am I getting out of it, and how much does that affect my past experiences?

What am I trying to solve as I move into the future?

I went to college with a woman who would buy clothes, wear them with the tags on, and return them within a week. This compulsive behavior pattern was a direct result of her low self-esteem from her relationship with her mother and a yearning for higher social status.

RELATIONSHIPS AND LOVE

Relationships and love go together in the same category of addiction because they both involve communication and interactions, which we consider a relationship. Relationships can be both friendships and moving beyond friendship, transitioning into romantic love.

In terms of both relationships and love, we tend to find the people we need to fill our voids. When you are with another individual—whether as a friend, spouse, or partner—you don't feel as alone.

In the times when you do feel alone, you may feel misunderstood or unheard, and you may not know how to cope on a day-to-day basis. When you feel alone, you tend to find people who support your ability to feel whole. The downside about this is that we tend to be attracted to people who are in similar situations at the same time as we are. You may question your current relationship or situation.

Imagine you are sad and depressed. It's easier to talk to someone else who is also sad and depressed. You feel like you are more understood. That's when you can go down the wrong path because you are feeding the negative part of yourself by choosing to be with someone you feel understands that negative side of you.

This occurs a lot in bars:

- You go out to a bar.
- You meet someone.
- You tell them about your bad day.
- They have had their own bad day.
- They tell you about it.

And now you're able to connect with each other.

You can also experience the opposite, where you meet someone who is very motivated, very goal-oriented, and very happy, and you're attracted to that.

That is the healthier way to go:

- Move toward people who are experiencing the opposite of what you're feeling, so they can help you get *out* of the situation.

- They can help you strategize a different way to move forward.

- That just breeds more happiness, and encourages you to be more orientated toward your goals in your own lifestyle.

The physiological and chemical responses within relationships fluctuate. An initial infatuation like an obsessive-compulsive disorder (OCD) can occur. This is why a breakup initiates a stalking behavior in some individuals.

Over the years in my practice, I've seen that love can manifest in different ways. When you first fall in love, there's a certain feeling you get. You're happy and everything is going well. Then, over time in your relationship, things don't seem to be as happy anymore. That feeling isn't there, and therefore you perceive your relationship as unhappy. But actually, it's just a shift in chemistry. Some people are addicted to that initial feeling connected to the OCD.

What are your OCD patterns?

Why do you feel you have them?

Are they linked to childhood connections with parents?

In choosing a partner or choosing friends, I like to use a metaphor presented to me at a wedding reception: I refer to an onion. You pick the perfect onion, but over time, the layers of the onion shed. As the layers shed, they expose feelings and just like an onion, when the core is exposed, it can make you cry.

In close long-term relationships:

- You get to the core of the individual.
- You learn more about your friend or partner.
- Your relationship can then flourish because it's not fake.

With text message, emails, and Internet communication, people are getting a false sense of love or belonging.

Facebook is a perfect example of filling emotional voids. When you connect on social media, you feel like you're not alone; you feel heard.

Understand that everyone has a different perception of what love feels like or how it is expressed. Expecting another to have a full understanding of your needs for love is like asking them to fix all of your past interactions with family and friends. That is not their job; it is yours.

FOOD, ALCOHOL, AND DRUGS

I group food, alcohol, and drug addictions together since each can directly alter brain chemistry related to the quantity and tolerance of a substance. Part of what creates substance addiction includes a shift in the quantities of receptor sites in the brain. This receptor site shift also causes changes in cognition. Your brain is genetically predisposed to the creation of more receptor sites; for instance, if a parent is alcoholic, you are more likely to have an addictive behavior pattern.

Upon stopping your drinking, you may follow what many alcoholics do: shift to soda, chips, orange juice, and all the sugary fillers that replace the sugar of the alcohol. This can occur with drugs as well because the sugar is still feeding that addiction pattern.

Because you are feeding the same brain-reward pathway with a different type of sugar, you are still stimulating that neuronal connection. In order to break that addiction completely, sugar cannot be a part of your diet *at all*. If you don't, it will make you more prone to holding on to that same addiction problem, but with a different substance. That is why alcoholics cannot take one sip of alcohol and a food addict cannot take one bite of sugar.

When you stop taking in the initial substance *and* limit your sugar intake, you biochemically manipulate your body to stop the cravings. When you do that, you'll be less apt to grab that alcohol or drug again. For better results, you must replace the substance with a goal to get to your vision.

Food has become an increasing problem because with marketing, visual stimuli draw on addictive behaviors. We eat things based on images or addictions to additives. So you go to the grocery store, and colors are good, or the language lures you in. The food you take into your body can change your chemistry and even make you more prone to believing the advertising.

Over time, the food can create an inflammatory response that will then generate a pain cycle within your body. This is a big problem. Pain is now typically controlled through medications, and currently, they are over-prescribed. The medications themselves can also be addictive.

Prescription opioids are becoming a gateway into the heavy drug addiction worlds. If you're overusing your pain medication, your doctor may decline to prescribe more. You may use them faster because you need more of the medication to relieve the pain. Your body has adapted to it and it takes greater amounts of the opiate to have the same effect. Your neurotransmitters are at maximum function, so taking a pill isn't giving you that same soothing feeling that your addiction craves.

Whatever the reason, if you find yourself without legal pain medication, that's when you could be most vulnerable to turning to drugs like cocaine and heroin. We don't look enough at our relationship to sugary foods and how that can really impact the whole pathway of biochemistry.

A patient of mine tried to stop drinking four years ago and began the habit of having Oreo cookies, juice, and toast in the morning. Then she'd have chicken and some veggies at lunch. She thought that that was a healthy shift. Once she started to eat all the foods listed above, she developed other medical complications. The minute she shifted away from sugary foods, she ended up trending back into the alcohol. No one had changed that biochemical pathway of her brain-reward system to handle the shift. This important piece is often lacking in patient care for addiction.

Addictive behaviors like those within the five categories described here can have very similar outcomes and processes. The key to overcoming any addiction is finding alternatives that will make you feel better. My work is helping people to change the reward system in the body through the neurotransmitters. You want a goal-directed reward system instead of a chemically directed reward system.

When you are able to achieve goal-directed reward systems, you can overcome your addictive behavior patterns:

- If you liked to go outside and bike just as much as you liked gambling, shopping, or your addictive substance or activity of choice, then that's what I would direct you to do more.

- If you were driven by money, we'd work on how to define a goal of what you need to do over the course of weeks and months to get to a better financial place.

- In relationships and love, everything you need is within you, and anything external is just a bonus. If we can stabilize you and have you be okay with yourself — love yourself — then you're probably not going to be as prone to trying to get your needs met through other substances, people, or through material items. You will be okay with just being with yourself; that's really the most important thing.

- In terms of food, alcohol, and drugs — whatever you're putting into your body — it all becomes your internal environment. It's up to you whether you are still going to McDonald's and being stimulated by the smell to eat fast food, or you stay out of those places and recognize that you feel healthier when you eat proteins, veggies, and fruits.

Your brain wants instant gratification, and because of technology, you're trying to feed that daily.

When we address addiction, these are key things that we look at:

- We look at your whole world and what you're doing to make an impact on your addiction systems.

- The body will still produce that pathway if you give it a behavior reward system.

- The chemical shifts in your body are still the same.

- Your body does not know what the addiction is; your body just knows the biochemical reaction that feeds the addiction.

CHAPTER **TWO**

Life

All living beings share the same capabilities preceding death:

- Growth
- Reproduction
- Functional activity
- Continual change

You never know what is going to happen. We're not all guaranteed to be here tomorrow.

Life can be expressed in five different ways:

- Expression of thought
- Expressions of genes
- Expressions of biochemical interactions
- Expressions of language
- Expressions of nature

These all impact us in certain ways that can take a positive or negative spin. A patient came into my office one day after being diagnosed with cancer. I asked her how she was coping.

She paused, looked me straight in the eye, and responded, "Life will go on without me."

I replied, "Yes, it will."

Then I explained to her that the life force was still within her at that moment. Her life force had been impacted by her own reality. Life is controlled by the state of our minds more than we realize. Her state of mind is her reality. At that point, her state of mind had become her disease, and her reality—what she wasn't aware of—was within her brain. Thoughts that we create in our brains can cause a disease state and suck the life out of cells, and eventually cause death.

Several patients of mine within the last few years have been misdiagnosed with a terminal cancer. Their reality in their mind changed upon hearing the diagnosis, and dis-ease set in.

When they went back for a follow-up, they were told that they had been misdiagnosed. Their state of mind had to make another shift. Our cells can't always do that. Their other healthcare providers had left them on their own to cope with the healing process of the biochemical shift that occurred within them. Radical changes, whether they are in state of mind, toxins, or food, can cause just as much cellular death as going into shock.

EXPRESSIONS OF THOUGHTS

B.J. Palmer said, "A liberation of a man's mind is from limitations of old principles to new principles."

That's a pretty key point when you look at expressions of thoughts, because you tend to get trapped in your own world—what I call the brain—and it is the perception of your reality that guides you.

The brain transmits information through dimensions, shading, and objects, and at each moment of thought, we believe it. We can talk ourselves into and out of anything. We create justification.

For example, you can tell yourself:

- *I can have ice cream today because I ate all my dinner.*
- *I can't go running today because I'm too tired.*
- *I can go buy a new car because I have met my goals and I deserve a reward.*

We don't realize that we can manifest changes within our brain, but they are our perception of what *we* think. Within the brain, we make choices every day. The quality of life is based on our choices. People can make a positive choice, and they get a positive outcome, or they make a negative choice and they get a negative outcome.

A positive choice when you're in high school might be not getting into a car with someone who is doing something illegal. A negative choice would be that you get in and then you participate in the same behavior as that person. They could be doing drugs, drinking alcohol, or getting into trouble. If you decide to go along, you may be making that choice to feel like you belong. You know it's wrong but you participate to fit in.

Instead, you need to really think for yourself.

What is it like to be with yourself?

Self-control actually comes from a *belief* system, not a *behavior* system. When you manifest reasons and justifications, you can talk yourself into and out of anything. We can look at self-control as an exercise for the brain.

Sometimes you might make choices based on your emotions. Your emotions can overtake your choices, when the brain is actually designed to *plan* them. Chapter Five explores emotions and how they can manifest and change brain thoughts.

When you think a stressful thought, you can actually change the substrates within your neurological system. Substrates are components that uptake serotonin. They uptake different chemicals; they're our feel-good chemicals. These substrates burn up in certain stressful situations. Research shows they are affected through the thought process. The more we are stressed, the more we want to feel good and the more we are prone to an addictive behavior to produce serotonin in the brain.

How can you break out of this cycle?

To get unstressed, you must have gratitude. When you

have gratitude, you can avoid an addictive behavior sooner. Stresses will be covered in Chapter Three.

EXPRESSIONS OF GENES

Organization occurs on a cellular level as well as throughout our environment. We can see this play out with our species and in our DNA. When the order is disrupted in DNA, chromosomal variations occur. One of the more common results of chromosomal variation that people are familiar with is Down syndrome.

There's a specific structure of atoms and molecules that have to be assembled for optimal functionality and adaptability. An example of this can be seen in the adaptability of your spinal column. The spinal column is made up of bones or vertebrae and discs of fluid that cushion and separate the vertebrae. The discs are made mostly of water. That is by design to allow for changes within the body. Adequate hydration is necessary to keep this system flowing in a healthy way.

If you do not drink enough water, if you allow yourself to become severely dehydrated, your body will actually pull water from the discs for other tasks. Over time, the discs shrink. Degenerative disc disease can set in as a result.

Another example of changes on a genetic level can be found in our food supply. Industrial agriculture has tried to address the need for abundant drought- and pest-resistant crops through the use of genetically modified organisms (GMOs). Genetic engineers combine desirable characteristics of one organism into another's DNA; for instance, they insert a bacterium into a plant so it will kill insects on its own rather than rely on an external pesticide. There is a lot of controversy over this practice because no one really knows the outcome over time. Many studies of animals fed exclusively GMO foods show organ damage over a short period of time. (See nongmoreport.com for more information.)

Our DNA and our cells were not made to handle many of the changes that humans have been exposed to. We may be producing more food initially using GMOs, but over the course of time, organic farming will produce more food.

These attempts at advancing our human lives are changing our genetic components, and many of them cause disruption to your system. Your food is supposed to feed your cells. When you put food in your body, it communicates with other cells, and through the communication, your body makes adaptations. If the food is not nutritive or has modified genes, when it gets into your body it's going to take on a negative cellular function. This is what happens with cells that become cancerous. They take on a replication pattern that is not normal.

The expression of genes can change through toxic

overload as well. One of the main organs of the body that rids toxins is the liver. The liver is dwindling in function, not only because of the toxins that we're putting into it, but also because of the inflammatory changes that are occurring with the change of genes within the body. When inflammation occurs in the intestinal tract, your body will try to pull the glutathione that's in the liver into the intestinal tract in order to decrease inflammation. We need glutathione to convert phase-one fat-soluble molecules to phase-two water-soluble molecules. If we don't have enough glutathione to make that happen, toxic buildup can occur and can create a lot of problems within our system. We refer to this as *fatty liver disease.*

EXPRESSIONS OF BIOCHEMICAL INTERACTIONS

Biochemical interactions occur because of positive and negative charges of atoms in the nuclei of your cells.

You can manipulate the charge of your cells through changing:

- Food
- Liquid
- Medication
- Chemistry
- Exposure to toxins

Let's look at how your biochemical interactions might change through food.

1. You bite food, take it into your mouth, and start chewing.

2. Digestion begins as your salivary glands release enzymes to break down the food.

3. When the food gets into your stomach, hydrochloric acid from the parietal cells continues the digestion.

4. If your stomach acid is compromised (e.g., because of sugary, processed foods or genetically modified foods), you're actually changing the state of the environment. Now that acidic environment in the stomach becomes more basic.

5. When the stomach acid becomes more basic, it doesn't break down food and food gets stuck. This can cause acid reflux or acid indigestion.

You might quickly pop a Tums antacid tablet in your mouth, which will then reduce the indigestion or acid reflux at that moment, but over time it shifts the hydrochloric acid function within the stomach and prevents the body from producing its normal amount. It will actually shift the chemistry so your food does not break down properly.

If your food is not breaking down properly, you may develop a nutritional depletion. Over time, the cells can lose their function. Sensitivities to food and leaky gut can occur in the absence of normal acidity for digestion.

We can also see nutrient depletion in the case of some medications. Pharmaceutical medications put into the body will change biochemical processes by shutting off enzyme function. When enzymes are shut off, nutrient depletion occurs, and chemistry shifts in the body causing a different problem. At that point, a patient would require a new medication for the new problem.

Biochemical interactions are affected by three main types of stress:

- Physical stress
- Chemical stress
- Emotional stress

Physical stress could be caused by a trauma, for instance:

- A fall
- A sports injury
- A car accident

Chemical stress can be influenced by our environment:

- Cleaning products
- Detergents
- Prescription and over-the-counter medications
- Herbal supplements taken inappropriately
- Emotions

Atoms have a tendency to attract each other when they have opposite charges and repel each other when they are the same. Attraction can result on a microscopic level from chemical changes brought about through ingesting food, drugs, or toxins; or it can be on more of a macroscopic level, like when we talk about interacting with people. Have you ever met an individual with whom you just "click"?

Our bodies experience significantly more stress than they did on average fifteen years ago. This is visible in looking at long-term impacts from trauma acquired in auto accidents. When we look at the stress that occurred in a body fifteen years ago, long-term problems would develop if impact occurred at thirty-five miles an hour or faster. Now we're seeing people having long-term effects with even ten-mile-an-hour impacts, because the body is already stressed.

Most people's systems are already inflamed, and once inflammation is present systemically, it's hard for your body to stop that process. It requires the right biochemical expression and interaction. You must target all areas, especially with autoimmune or neurological diseases.

One of the best ways to reduce emotional stress is to cultivate gratitude. When you have gratitude, you cannot be stressed on a cellular level. There's a great book called *The Five Minute Journal*. The author suggests waking up in the morning, being thankful, and writing down what you're grateful for. In the evening, reflect on the day, remember what you are grateful for, and write it down. This simple act will have a big impact on your cellular function. You don't want cells that are stressed. Stressed cells make people sick and dis-eased. Another book that helps people express gratitude is *The Magic* by Rhonda Byrne.

To help reduce emotional stress, choose to be with people who make you *feel* better, not the ones who only make you *look* better. There's a difference.

You want to be around people who:

- Support you
- Bring you to another level
- Are there for you
- Promote happiness
- Promote gratitude

These are the ones who will help you the most.

EXPRESSIONS OF LANGUAGE

Language can also be expressed through interactive behavior patterns with animals and humans on a cellular level. You can transmit information from one individual to another, one cell to another.

Expressions of language include:

- Words
- Gestures
- Movements
- Sound

Some things can be silent, and some things can have noise. You can use various ideas to communicate as long as the other person receives the information.

Your body and brain receive and deliver information differently. Think of the childhood game of Telephone, in which one person whispers a message to the next in a circle. That person whispers to the next until the message has made it all the way around the circle. By the time the message gets to the end, it's usually not the same. Small variations between whisperers along the way add up because of how we receive and deliver information.

At orientation for the ALIVE program, we show participants an image and ask them to write down the first four things that they see in that image. One couple participating in the program had communication problems. The woman reported that they would get into arguments often, and at the end of the argument, they would both realize they were talking about the same thing. I asked them both to respond to the image, to write down the first four things that came to mind.

The man listed the objects from back to front, and the woman listed the objects from front to back. The information they put on their pieces of paper was identical. The difference was that he saw the world from far to near, and she saw near to far. So although they had the same information, because they started at different ends of the spectrum, they weren't able to communicate freely. It had created a lot of turmoil within their relationship.

Finding different ways to communicate with people is another important way to alleviate stress on your system.

EXPRESSIONS OF NATURE

When considering expressions of nature, I like to use the five elements from several traditions:

- Fire
- Earth
- Metal
- Water
- Wood

These elements have different meanings and they are associated with seasonal changes:

- Wood is associated with spring.
- Fire is associated with summer.
- Earth corresponds with late summer.
- Metal corresponds with autumn.
- Water corresponds with winter.

The five elements or components of nature also correlate with structures and systems within your body:

- Water relates to your kidneys.
- Metal relates to your lungs and large intestines.
- Earth relates to your spleen and stomach.

- Fire relates to your heart and small intestines.
- Wood relates to your liver and gall bladder.

How do the elements interact?

If you haven't drunk enough water, for example, your kidneys are going to be affected. If you drink too much water late in the evening, you are going to be up in the night urinating because you're flushing out your kidneys.

What is the relationship between the organs in your body and their functions?

How do they shift based on what you do and the time of year?

In springtime, for example, you might have seasonal allergies.

Have you ever wondered why you have a seasonal allergy?

Some people are tested for external, environmental sources, but no one ever thinks about the connection to their organs or the connection to their emotions.

You may be surprised to learn that there is a connection between the liver and allergies. If you have seasonal allergies, we might put you on a liver cleanse to help deal with or manage or remove the allergic stimulus within your system.

In autumn, you are transitioning into winter. You may

develop a cold. You have a stuffy nose and then the congestion settles into your lungs. This isn't by chance; this is all by design.

You need to try to understand how your organs are relating to what's going on in the environment. If you can do this, then you can begin the process of healing dis-eases within the system.

Another correlation to the expressions of nature is through the five tastes.

Salty: When you crave salty foods, it's because your body is trying to retain water. The flavor of salt is associated with the water element and winter.

Spicy: Spicy is associated with the metal element, which corresponds with autumn. In autumn, you typically will have nasal congestion and lung problems. Spicy food clears out your sinuses.

Sweet: Late summer, which corresponds with earth, has to do with sweet foods. Sweet foods can feed the earth at late summer, and they are correlated with the spleen. The spleen is our immune system, so when our immune system is down, we feel weak. When we feel weak, we're more prone to having sugar, because that gives us more energy.

Bitter: In the summer, it's typically hot. People will tend toward bitter foods. We don't really consume a lot of bitter foods these days. Recent brain research has found there's a cranial nerve in your brain stem that is associated with bitter flavors. If you do not experience bitter tastes — like fennel, for example — then the cranial nerve will not be as stimulated.

Umami: This savory taste activates glutamate, a neurotransmitter used in cellular metabolism. The flavor of umami is associated with spring, which is the cleansing time.

Expressions of nature can be very healing and provide another avenue toward optimal cellular function, externally and internally.

Life is challenging to a lot of people. Challenges begin when you are in the womb. You have to look at the very beginning of development to give the body what it needs. Then the challenge is to keep that going as you grow and mature.

Focus on what's important for taking care of your body, and not what food or medication is easier to grab because of our fast-paced society. We are depleting our nutritional stores over time, and causing a lot of increased diseases as a result.

Just look at the average birth weights of babies. Newborns have been getting progressively larger. The average weight at birth has gone from six pounds to nine pounds. As the size of your infant increases, it is more challenging for you to give birth naturally, without intervention. More protein, up to 80–150 grams of protein a day, can keep the birth weight down. But we don't really educate our mothers about proper nutrition.

We are a sugar-loading society, and the more sugar you have in your system, the more prone you are to having bigger babies. The bigger your babies, the more prone they are to neurological impacts on the healthy function of cells.

If we are going to maintain optimal expressions of our cells through time, we've got to get back to basic needs and principles.

CHAPTER THREE

Innate Intelligence

Innate intelligence is a chiropractic term that was first coined by Daniel David Palmer, who was the founder of chiropractic. We use this term for the organizing properties of living things. B.J. Palmer's *thirty-three chiropractic principles* explain the adaptation of forces we call innate intelligence in relation to cellular matter.

The Universal Laws are based on physiology and physics. When you try to change the mechanisms or impact of cells or tissues — because the human race is trying to invent the next best cleaning product, or the next best computer, or cell phone — then you disrupt the structure and balance of molecules and cells.

Many people are still unaware that everything in the body — the function of every cell, tissue, organ, and system of the body — is controlled by the nervous system. Chiropractic was designed to help prevent the nervous system's dysfunction. We chiropractors typically work within five different categories to accomplish an organized matter.

The five categories are:

- Histopathology

- Kinesiopathology
- Pathophysiology
- Myopathology
- Neuropathophysiology

What follows is a description of each category, why it's important, and how it relates to the healing of any disease and function of the body.

HISTOPATHOLOGY

Histopathology is the study of abnormal tissue function. Abnormal tissue function can come from a variety of different impacts. The first one is disc malfunction.

Discs are between the vertebrae of the spinal column. They are designed to promote a cushion and allow proper movement between the vertebrae. The disc has a blood supply only on the outside, and the inside is mainly composed of water. If injured, the disc takes a long time to heal because the blood supply is on the outside only.

Another kind of tissue makes up your ligaments. They occur along the spinal column among other joints in the body and provide a different kinds of flexibility. Nutritional deficiencies in our system will change the elasticity of ligaments. Those changes may be a tightening or a release — more flexibility within the spine — that might not be a good component for a healthy individual.

The immune system is highly dependent upon healthy tissue and cell function. When your body is continually challenged on a cellular level, your immune system kicks in to try to heal that area. If the body doesn't have the right chemical components to heal that area, then over time your immune system becomes weaker and weaker. Then the metabolic function cells will change.

Metabolic functions of cells can also change due to the toxins within our environment. Chemical changes are a big concern. When we use cleaning products or make plastics, or interact daily with those chemicals—paints, solvents, carpet components that release a gas or give off a chemical substance that we breathe—they can create a change in metabolic function.

The other main component that is changing cellular function at this time is the use of cell phones and Internet. There are positive and negative charges within your system. Different forms of wavelengths come in from sources like wifi hot spots or cellular transmission. They hit your cells and change the interactions between your cells at different levels. When this occurs, the functionality of the cell will change. Over time, this can cause either cell death or added growth within your system, like a tumor or a cyst within the body.

A device called a *Pulsed Electromagnetic Field* (PEMF) *Machine* is a very effective tool to improve cellular function, metabolism, and detoxification. It helps cells return to a normal state. A study compared blood samples from an individual prior to and after being put on a PEMF machine. Before the session, the patient's blood cells were smaller and stagnant, not moving. After a session of three to five minutes, the cells were bigger and moving.

When blood cells are bigger and moving, they're able to take in more oxygen and transport oxygen in the body more efficiently. They can provide the cellular nutrition that is needed to maintain the normal cell function, instead of the diseased cell function.

KINESIOPATHOLOGY

Kinesiopathology is the study of atypical positioning or abnormal motion of vertebrae. The relationship of vertebrae can change pressure loads on the spine over time and develop restrictive patterns. This can cause a lot of irritation within the body on a cellular level. There are a couple of different categories that can cause malpositioning or abnormal motion within the spinal column.

Physical Trauma

Physical trauma occurs from injuries, such as those sustained in sports, car accidents, falls, or domestic abuse.

When someone has a car accident and they are in a head-on collision, the impact that occurs—with a forward force in the cervical neck region—can create an abnormality within the body. Sometimes, if the impact is great enough, one vertebra can jump over another and cause a spinal cord injury, or even death at that time. As stated in the previous chapter, people are now experiencing long-term trauma from even low-force impacts because we are all inflamed and our cells aren't functioning as they should be.

Repetitive Motion Trauma

Repetitive motion trauma can develop from gardening, computer workstations, using a mouse, sitting at a desk all day, leaning forward, or staying in one position. It's always good to try to get up and move every twenty to thirty minutes, or even change your activity if you can. You might want to garden first, then stack some wood, then garden again. That will help your body avoid the repetitive motion pattern that occurs.

Poor Sleeping Habits

Many people don't realize that their bed may change the pressure loads on the spine and can cause them a lot of distress at night, especially in the cervical region. You might have a tendency to move pillows in certain directions or ways. This makes you jam the facet joints of the spine, which can cause a lot of inflammation. The facet joints of the spine are in the back, and they allow for proper motion and rotation. Sleep habits can also be affected by your laundry detergent and dryer sheets. Dryer sheets are actually linked to sudden infant death syndrome (SIDS).

Stress

Both chemical and emotional stress can affect the motion or positioning of your spine. Emotions can impact your spinal column and your nervous system. When you are stressed, you nervous system is going to be stressed. As your nervous system increases the stress load, then it's going to change the position or fixate a position. Chemicals within the bed sheets or our clothing can actually create a stress on our nervous system, and cause neurological problems. Chemical stressors can also be medications, food, liquids, and environmental factors such as acid rain, which we aren't even aware of.

Birth

The last category that can change the spinal column is the birthing process. One of my newest patients was a breech baby. Medical staff attending the birth tried to turn the baby before doing a C-section. When they pulled the baby out, they positioned the baby so her head was stuck to the side. Until getting adjusted, the baby was unable to move her head to the right, and she was having problems breastfeeding and digesting. We don't always realize the impact of changing the position of the vertebrae, and how that can affect our disease state.

PATHOPHYSIOLOGY

Pathophysiology is the study of the abnormal functions of the spine and body, such as cellular changes, structural changes in the spinal column, bone spurs, spinal decay, or fusion of the joints. It can involve calcium deposits or soft tissue changes. These are all indications of changes within the spine. X-rays can help in diagnosing bone spurs or bony protrusions usually in the anterior aspect of the vertebrae. They can curl around the disc in a protective manner. If this occurs at the three vertebral bodies, then it's an indication that the person has a condition called *diffuse idiopathic skeletal hyperostosis (DISH)*. This condition is usually linked to diabetes or sugar-handling problems. It's just one way to diagnose what's happening in the system.

Spinal decay can be in the form of *osteopenia* or *osteoporosis*, which is usually present because the body is trying to use calcium in another place. Again, the body has the innate intelligence and the adaptability to try to keep itself well, so it will pull calcium from the bone to try to solve a problem in a different place. That's why osteopenia and eventually osteoporosis occurs.

If children experience pain when teething, it can be because they don't have enough calcium in their system. That's what causes tooth pain; you need calcium to make bone, and your tooth is a bone. Kids don't always have enough resources to build bone.

As the spine degenerates, it puts pressure on the nerves. The nerves control the function of all the organs themselves. Organs can malfunction. As an example, you could have a liver that is not functioning due to pressure on the nerve that is causing a transmission problem. It prevents the body from functioning appropriately.

Many older women have urinary incontinence. It may be passed off as a typical symptom of aging, when it's usually due to years of spinal pressure changes on a nerve that causes a malfunction over time. Many women have been told that it's because they had a child and they didn't do enough Kegel exercises, but it's really due to spinal changes that create a malfunction in the nervous system.

MYOPATHOLOGY

Myopathology is the study of the muscles and their role in supporting the spine. Abnormal muscle function can contribute to the disease of the body. When muscles are abnormal, they are weakened. You might experience this as atrophy, spasms, or tight muscles.

Two years ago, a patient came in with a DNA-malfunctioning disease that created such tightness in his muscles that at times he could not walk. When I took an X-ray of his spine, I discovered that his C1 and occipital vertebra—the skull bone—were fused together. When they are fused, proper nerve transmissions cannot occur to create proper muscle movements. Over time, your body will just contract inside so your hands, legs, and feet come up toward the core of your body. The more this patient tried to walk standing up, the more pain he had.

The nerves can really affect muscle control, weakness, and atrophy. Sometimes there is a disc problem in the lower spine and if a nerve is injured, it prevents you from moving your foot or walking. Muscles can change size, as when unused over time and they shrink or atrophy.

If you don't take care of the restriction patterns of the spine that we call *subluxations*, you are more prone to having scar tissue and adhesions build up within the spine. That can create a lot of stiffness and inability to move as well. The less movement you make, the more pressure on the nervous system. The more pressure, the more potential there is for any other part of the system to malfunction, whether it's your blood pressure or your organ function. It depends on what level of the vertebrae supports that region of the body. For instance, your C6, C7, and T1 vertebrae all help the control of sugar handling within the system. You create a feedback loop in which you are eating sugar, sugar then affects the spinal column and causes a subluxation; or, the subluxation can cause the inability to regulate sugar appropriately.

Muscles are important because you use them to move. Muscles that contain a toxic load can be painful.

There's a disorder called *fibromyalgia,* but in my professional opinion, fibromyalgia is secondary — more symptomatic of another condition than a disorder on its own. We need to look more at how to make a shift relative to internal, inflammatory disease within the system.

NEUROPATHOPHYSIOLOGY

Neuropathophysiology is the study of nerve connections within the body. Nerve connections can transport information like cellular function. They also affect our behavior, as discussed in the first chapter. Basic nerve transmission runs from the brain down the spinal column into the periphery. Improper function can cause changes within the tissues, organs, and systems.

Too much transmission, which is overstimulation, can create a hyperactivity within the cell function. This can lead to seizures. One patients had an oversensitivity such that any time she bumped into something, it would create a seizure-like reaction and cause her to drop to the ground. As we started working with her spine, and slowly working with the brain cells to reconnect the neuropathophysiology, she experienced less dramatic reactions to bumping into things.

The neurons are vital to every function of the body. They contain your innate intelligence. Your body has the ability to do things without even thinking about it.

Your innate intelligence governs things you don't make a decision about:

- Your heart rate
- Circulating blood to your lungs to oxygenate your blood
- Adapting to a change in temperature

Another example is when elastic, such as at the waistband or the top of your socks, creates an indentation in your skin. Then you take the band off and your skin returns to its regular shape. We call this *hysteresis*. Your body adapts to that change, and you don't think about that adaptation.

Innate intelligence is designed to keep your body to a functioning state, and keep your body well. It needs to do that with the perfect environment, as much as possible.

What is the perfect environment?

One in which your body has what it needs:

- Enough water
- Enough nutrients
- No chemicals
- No toxins
- Good digestion

Your innate intelligence will help you — no matter what — through a functioning state, through a healthy state, through a diseased state. But it will do better when you give your body what it needs, and your cells will be able to regenerate if your body has the proper chemical cellular reactions within it.

The nervous system regulates everything. You have to consider all avenues in order to maintain a healthier body. With our toxic environment and the dis-eased trend that we're taking within the healthcare system, we are going to have to start looking at how we are made, how the cells function, and how we get them well, instead of grabbing the next pill to change the symptom and mask the dis-ease.

If you're on blood pressure meds, and you don't take the pill the next day, will your blood pressure go up?

If the answer is yes, you haven't addressed the cause of the blood pressure. You're not fixing the main cause of the problem. In order to get your innate intelligence to function appropriately, you have to start looking at the problem.

What is the cause of the illness?

When we get back to a healthcare system that actually looks at preventative care, looking at how cells function and what they need, then more people will be well and fewer people will be in a dis-eased state.

CHAPTER FOUR

Vision

A successful person attains success by never losing track of the vision. An unsuccessful person sees the obstacles along the way as burdens that may take longer to overcome. Failure comes from imagined impossibilities.

Your vision helps you aspire to be better and do better, not just for yourself, but also for the people around you. You can also think of vision as setting goals.

Goals can be short-term and long-term, set as an individual or as a group. There's a cost-benefit relationship that occurs when you set goals. That has a critical value and offers vitality to each individual on a neurological and cellular level.

To be able to make a shift in brain chemistry from a dis-eased state to one of wellness, you need to set goals and find your motivation in one of the five categories:

- Achievement
- Society
- Incentives
- Fear
- Change

Where you are right now and where you want to be depends somewhat on how you feel about yourself. But it is also affected by how you perceive the world and how the world perceives you. There's an interesting connection between the neurological pathways created by setting your goals and the ones affected by addiction (as described in the first chapter).

MOTIVATION FROM ACHIEVEMENT

Achievement motivation is related to setting a vision or a goal with a specific outcome in mind. For instance, you want to learn how to ski. Your achievement is that you want to get to the bottom of the hill without falling. Another example of achievement motivation would be going to school with the goal of receiving a diploma.

Achievement motivation usually requires a day-in, day-out follow-through of practice, reading, and education to get from one goal to another. You also typically complete a series of steps to arrive at your goal. In the skiing example, maybe you'd start by learning how to put on your gear. Then you'd learn to ride the chair lift. You can't learn it all in one step. It takes several times to try to achieve this goal. Achievement motivation usually requires a lot of time and effort over a set length of time.

MOTIVATION FROM SOCIETY

Motivation by society can be a good thing, but it can also be a big challenge.

Should you care what people think of you?

Societal motivation includes taking in messages from media like television and advertising and then assessing what they are doing to us as individuals. Consider weight gain or loss. You're constantly flooded with messages of the next best thing to control your weight. You are exposed to images of tiny models, so you are trained to think that smaller is more desirable. You're actually creating false ideas within your mind because of society's marketing.

Feeling motivated by society can be a negative situation. You could develop an eating disorder, for example, because you believe that you have to be tinier to match the images on TV. Societal motivation can be a positive circumstance, in which you look at the TV and you realize that you should have some weight loss because your current heavier weight is unhealthy and puts stress on your heart.

Here's one of the ways that societal motivation can shift our thoughts and thought patterns. A common belief is that you need a degree to be successful in society, but many highly successful individuals never graduated high school. They are still highly motivated and productive within our society. Some people who never graduated are inventors, entrepreneurs, or successful business owners.

Schooling does not mean that you are guaranteed to have a job, and not going to school doesn't mean that you are guaranteed not to be successful. I'm not promoting one way over the other; I am just showing the different ways that people can perceive a motivation or a vision.

MOTIVATION FROM INCENTIVES

Incentives can come in the form of monetary bonus, special activities, or opportunities. In a job, perhaps if you complete a task, you're rewarded with a bonus. A child might gain reward by doing chores; if you took out the trash on a Saturday morning, you were allowed to go out with friends that afternoon.

Depending on what age group we're looking at or what the incentive is, people have the ability to rationalize why they should complete a goal or a vision to then get a different outcome.

MOTIVATION FROM FEAR

Our culture uses fear as motivation frequently.

Children are told, "If you do this, then you're not going to be able to have that."

You may use your child's fear of making you angry to change their behavior. If you want a different outcome, if you want to help your children to the next phase, you actually just need to love them, not make them afraid.

Fear can have a huge impact on the function of organs. In the next chapter on emotions, you'll see how fear can change the health of an organ. Fear creates disease.

Fear can be present in a relationship with a dominating person. The non-dominating partner is unable to live their daily life, fearing that there will be ramifications to doing what they're doing. A situation like this affects your ability to make daily choices.

Are you making your choice because of the present, based on what's inside of you, or is your choice based on past experiences?

You may be making choices according to how you were raised, and the fears that your parents may have instilled in you. One of the examples that we see often is in parents coping with their pregnant teenager. The teenage child makes her choice about whether to continue or terminate the pregnancy based on parental guidance and what she fears.

Some partners live in fear of abuse. A man or a woman may fear either leaving their house or doing a certain task because of past verbal or physical abuse. Often these individuals have learned not to show what's going on in the household, so it's difficult to know what's happening behind closed doors.

Fear of illness can motivate us as well. If you were afraid that excess weight would cause a heart attack, it could motivate you to lose the excess. The fear of dying from cancer might motivate you to grasp at any solution to enhance longevity.

MOTIVATION FROM CHANGE

Some people love change, and other people don't like it at all. Change is interesting. You may know that you have to make a change in your lifestyle — maybe in how you interact with people — but change is hard. Change means that you have to do work. It means that you are outwardly admitting that something you are doing at that time is not working, is not correct, or could be better if you did it some other way. Change is a motivational factor that is harder for some people to understand.

People sometimes avoid the persuasion to change because they don't want to admit to any inadequacies within their daily life or their personal life. In your mind, you are consciously and unconsciously admitting to not doing something correctly. It is the hardest category for people to overcome at times.

A common saying is that the definition of *insanity* is doing the same thing over and over again but expecting different results.

Committing to making a change means that you are admitting that what you're doing or how you're living is not right. If you want to make a shift in your chemistry or your lifestyle, you have to do something differently. If not, according to that popular quote, you'd be considered insane for repeating the same actions over and over again but expecting different results.

When I present a lecture or seminar, there is always a

woman or man who is five-foot-five and 300 pounds who attends and listens. Either they don't recognize that they need to make a change, or they *do* recognize that they need to make a change, but they're not willing or able to put in the time and the effort that's needed to make that shift.

I often wonder how it is that they know they are the ones who need to be at these seminars, but they're not willing to or able to make that shift and get out of the routine that they're in. Not all individuals who are overweight have an eating problem. They might have a hormonal problem or an emotional problem that is causing their system to maintain their current weight.

Remember some of the ways to replace the same chemical changes that occur through addictive behaviors with healthy behaviors:

- Making a change in your internal biochemistry
- Understanding how you perceive the world
- Figuring out what motivates you
- Discovering what makes you happy

The connection between having a vision and setting daily, weekly, monthly, or yearly goals will help you be a better, more satisfied person. It will also help the people around you. You'll be more productive. Your cells will be healthier. If you have any of the addiction problems in the five categories mentioned earlier, having a concrete goal while using a different motivation strategy will give your neuronal pathways the ability to make a shift. You will be less likely to return to addictive habits.

Goals are steppingstones to visions.

What are your goals?

What is your vision?

CHAPTER **FIVE**

Emotions

Every emotion has a physiological source and response. Emotions are expressed within our bodies based on how we view or perceive the world.

We perceive the world through our:

- Wisdom
- Knowledge
- Moral expressions
- Values

Emotions are expressions of our neurological coping skills. Think long and hard enough about something and you can change the physical response within your body. You can think about a car cutting you off on the highway, almost causing an accident, and your blood pressure will rise. You can worry about where your children are, when they were supposed to be home by a certain time and have not called, and create anxiety.

Your brain has been trained throughout your life to react in a certain way based on:

- Your surroundings
- Your upbringing
- How well you digest nutrients

- Exposure to toxins in food (e.g., sugar)
- Exposure to environmental toxins

An emotion can cause a change in the function of an organ, or an organ can cause changes in emotions. This feedback loop has an impact on our coping skills. Your coping skills and neuronal connections change due to the impact of physiological processes. This is why a patient can participate in a structured detoxification program and—after only a week—report being better able to cope with the stress of life.

One patient came into our facility after seven days of detoxing and said, "Someone just cut me off. A week ago, I would have reacted with cuss words, and it would have ruined my day. Today, I smiled and said, 'Enjoy your day! This is your problem, not mine.'"

There are five major emotional categories that have the biggest impact on our physiological responses.

ANGER

The emotion anger is linked to the liver and gall bladder. To help you understand this concept a little bit more, let's look at the function of the liver and the gall bladder. The gall bladder sits on the liver and stores and concentrates a digestive enzyme that the liver makes called bile. The liver is a toxic waste station that filters blood, metabolizes nutrients, detoxifies harmful substances, makes blood-clotting proteins, produces cholesterol, and performs other vital functions.

When you feel angry, you directly impact liver function. The longer the emotion has been present, the more diseased the organ function will be. If you have a lot of unresolved anger, you are more prone to having alcohol, drug, or food addictions.

The loop is created by a toxic overload in food chemistry. For instance, if you are addicted to alcohol or food, then you're going to be prone to having more anger or emotional problems.

Is it the anger causing your liver to malfunction, or is it the liver malfunction causing the anger?

Symptoms associated with liver distress include:

- Headaches
- Knee pain
- Unexplainable strokes
- Seizures
- Dizziness
- Blurred vision
- Indigestion
- Skin disorders

The liver can affect the gall bladder and as a result, your ability to think straight.

A patient might say, "I'm so angry I can't even think."

The liver will also have an impact on the kidneys. If you have experienced emotional or physical abuse as a child, you are more prone to having liver problems.

GRIEF

Grief is associated with the large intestines and the lungs. Grief is also associated with the metal element. Grief often arises when people experience death in a family. This is why you are more prone to getting sick around the time that a death occurs.

Some diseases of the lungs are:

- Chronic obstructive pulmonary disorder (COPD)
- Asthma
- Emphysema

If you have unresolved grief, you are prone to having functional problems within the lungs. There is usually an emotional link to these diseases due to grief that you haven't resolved; it could be because of a death or an event.

Confidence is also associated with the lungs. If you lack confidence, you're going to show more signs of being prone to lung problems like asthma. If you have problems with grief, you are also more prone to smoking tobacco or marijuana. Because you haven't fed the emotion, you're now feeding that lung capacity. Even though it's in a negative way, it's still a way that you're feeding into the system.

The lungs are important because they process the oxygen we breathe, and oxygen is needed for all cellular functions. If you're breathing inappropriately due to asthma or COPD, then the alveolar sacs in the lungs aren't pulling in enough oxygen, and they're not releasing enough carbon dioxide into the air. Over time, this can feel very constricting to people.

FEAR, GUILT, AND JEALOUSY

Fear, guilt, and jealousy are linked to the kidney and bladder. Fear can enter in two different ways. It can come in with the water element, through the kidneys and liver. It can also manifest within the gall bladder.

Your kidneys excrete water. Water is needed to help all cells work properly. When you haven't been drinking enough water, you're prone to eating salty foods. If you eat a lot of salty foods, then you're going to hold on to more water. Your kidneys will not be able to do the work they need to do.

You need water for many systems in the body:

- Water prevents you from dehydrating.
- Water keeps the brain working well.
- Water prevents disc degeneration in the spine.
- Water is needed for peristalsis (movement of food through the digestive tract).
- Water promotes homeostasis.

Not drinking enough water can especially affect digestion. If you don't have enough water, your intestines will not be able to push the food and wastes through. As the food builds up on the out-pouches of the intestinal wall, it can ferment, causing disease on the outside of the wall and changes in cell function and structure. Because of deterioration in the intestinal wall over time, bigger molecules can get stuck in spaces where only little molecules should have been.

WORRY

Worry is connected to the spleen and stomach. It's associated with the element of earth. Many people know that if you're more stressed or worried, you're going to be prone to ulcers. That's because the stomach is in charge of breaking down food. It's second after the salivary glands in the sequence of the digestive system.

The stomach is where you begin assimilating nutrients. It is also where we assimilate life experiences, through the earth component of the five elements. Overwhelming life experiences can impact our stomach and spleen. The stomach then will have low hydrochloric acid (HCL) and food won't break down food as it's supposed to. When the food doesn't break down, it sits there, and the acid of the stomach will actually increase. The acid of the stomach increases and this is what causes the ulcers.

The medical world will typically suggest taking a Tums to calm the increase in stomach acid. They should instead prescribe an alternative, apple cider vinegar, to get the chemistry of the stomach back to normal, so the food can break down appropriately. This can be debilitating for some people.

Just as with the feedback loop between anger and the liver, worry and the stomach can loop into a cycle. Worry can affect the stomach or, if your stomach's not breaking food down, that can cause you to worry.

JOY AND SADNESS

Joy and sadness are linked to love, which is linked to the heart. In the heart area of the body, you build upon relationships to generate love, trust, and honesty. Your ability to do this is directly linked to how you were raised when you were a kid.

How did your parents, family members, and the surrounding people imprint on your nervous system?

If you see your parents manipulate and steal, you'll follow in their footsteps unless you learn from someone else that this is a wrong behavior pattern. Typically, at a young age, you start to observe how other people behave (such as when you visit a friend's house) and you begin to wonder why. This is the first step to questioning what's right or what's wrong.

Some people never have exposure to a different lifestyle, so they see only what they're raised with, and then they repeat those actions. Other people question the differences they see between their parents and other people.

When you start to put things together about the world, when you start making sense of it, you can change behavior patterns. Even now you can change how you look at the world and how you treat people, based on what they see other people doing. You can depict in your mind what is right and what is wrong.

Symptoms of difficulties with the heart include:

- Palpitations
- Insomnia
- Anxiety
- Emotional imbalances

Triggers can have an impact on the heart based on the neuronal pathways you created in childhood.

Remember the onion in the garden from Chapter One?

In a new relationship, everything is happy; everything is good. The new relationship feeds the heart and makes us happy. As we get deeper into the relationship, we learn more about our mate. This is where the onion effect comes in: you learn more about someone and yourself, like you see more of the core of the onion as it sheds its layers. As you shed the layers, things might not be as happy.

Some people really like the feeling of this happiness in a new relationship, so they're addicted to behaviors that will feed this emotional need. One patient was addicted to that feeling, so he would have relationships via email, to feed the heart area for that pathway. It was an addictive behavior that he didn't understand until he participated in our program. Then he was able to understand that it came from the emotional connection to how he was raised, what was going on when he was a child. He could see that it manifested as an addiction as he got older.

You also may experience jealousy, regret, and disappointment, if your heart has been *broken*. The heart hasn't really been broken, it's just that the heart chemistry has changed, so instead of joy coming out and being expressed neurologically, sadness comes out and expresses itself neurologically.

These emotions also connect with the small intestine, where you upload nutrients. If you are feeling sad, you're not going to upload nutrients as effectively. This can create a lot of problems within your system.

Eating the right foods can make you happy. When you feel that your heart has been broken, you might turn to food to soothe yourself. Food feeds the small intestine, which then feeds the heart, which then makes us happy. You can see how the connection between an emotion and the function of an organ can really have a positive or negative impact depending on where we are in life.

If you have a food addiction, is the food addiction coming from an emotional need, or is it coming from an organ insufficiency, malfunction, or disease?

Recently, one of my patients was dealing with liver toxic overload. The liver gives feedback to the small intestines. If you take in a sugary food, the liver doesn't have to produce the same amount of bile for the gall bladder. The gall bladder spits that unneeded bile into the stomach and the small intestines to be broken down. If you're eating sugar, your liver doesn't have to work as hard; but if you're eating a protein, your liver will have to work harder to assist in the breakdown of that protein.

This individual had been having some liver problems that were undiagnosed. She was eating more sugary foods and had caused a sugar addiction within her system. You can have a direct relationship with one organ that affects another area of the body, whether it's an organ, function, or emotion.

When analyzing what effects are going on within a diseased or a healthy system, we have to look at your ability to handle organ functions *and* emotions. Because there's a feedback loop that occurs biochemically, we have the ability to help you get over certain challenges in life and to change triggers within your system, based on this relationship between emotions and organ function. If you have coping skills in one area, we can manipulate an organ to actually help you overcome an emotion. We can also manipulate an emotion to help you overcome an organ function.

Simply drinking a number of ounces of water

equivalent to half the number of pounds of your body weight (e.g., 75 ounces of water for 150 pounds), you help your body and your cells to handle emotional instabilities. We live in a society where we are go-go-go-go-go all the time, and not enough people slow down. It's having a huge impact on our emotional state as a culture. We focus on instant gratification because we are not feeding ourselves enough in a soulful and emotional way. We are not looking at the biochemical relationship between the functionality of one entity and how it relates to another.

When we look and reflect on each individual's diseased state, we see what emotions are present, how they impact the system, how they impact us cellularly, and how we can make changes to help our bodies get to a better place.

Conclusion

Each of the five components that we've talked about in the ALIVE program take time for you to process. Look at how different components of each category apply to your own life.

What daily steps and weekly steps can you make to change cellular function within your body?

Your cells didn't become dis-eased in a day, and they're not going to become healthy in a day. Understand that as with any process in life, there is a time component. Do the best that you can to target areas you know you can change initially. Seek guidance for the others that you know need to change, but you don't know how to change within the parameters of your own lifestyle.

What resources are available within your community?

You may find a variety of helpers:

- Health coaches
- Life coaches
- Psychiatrists
- Psychologists
- Chiropractors
- Hypnotherapists
- Naturopaths
- Functional medicine MDs

They can help you find different strategies. There are emotional release techniques that can work with some of these components. Sometimes you just need to sit down, be with yourself, recognize which components you have worked on, which ones you are avoiding, and why, and try to understand yourself.

I think we don't take enough time to understand ourselves. We're bombarded with a lot of neuronal stimuli on a daily basis. Our brains are preoccupied. We don't take the time to really reflect to see how these methods can apply. Try meditation to get these components to resonate together, and find out what works for you. Everyone is different. Some people learn and change using visuals, while some learn and change through audio input. It's all about finding the best tool to help you through each component.

My gift to my readers is life! Enjoy the challenge of changing your thoughts, your emotions, your visions, and your expression of life, because we get only one body and one mind. We seem to take that for granted.

Please visit our website at www.backtolifenh.com and click on "A.L.I.V.E." You'll find tools and techniques to start healing yourself to target the different categories for cellular function.

Enjoy life! Be happy about yourself. Be committed to yourself. Know that you're the most important person on this earth. Stop sabotaging yourself. You are in control of your destiny.

Next Steps

Are you ready to take action?

Is your past acting as gravity, weighing you down?

Take the first step to making a change today.

Some people will read this book, understand all the concepts, and be able to apply them to their own lives effectively.

Other people will have an understanding of parts of it, but will not be able to apply it in a way to make the changes they need toward wellness.

If you want to make a change and this program resonates with you, you can go to our website, www. backtolifenh.com, and sign up for a complimentary thirty-minute phone consult on your health, needs, and concerns. One of our staff members will guide you through the process to create a customized ALIVE program designed specifically for you.

Bring this book with you to your consultation and you'll be eligible for a $200.00 additional discount on your customized ALIVE program!

About the Author

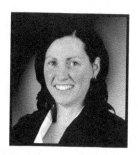

Dr. Stephanie J. Clark is a 2004 graduate of Palmer College of Chiropractic. She obtained a degree in Sports and Exercise Science with concentration in Movement Therapy and a minor in Psychology from Stetson University in 1997. While at Stetson, she studied the effects of cellular health in relationship to time of day.

Dr. Clark helped start a physical therapy unit in a whole-health practice in DeLand, Florida, where she worked under Dr. Stephen Hayman and Dr. Randall Timko. She moved to New Hampshire and continued her studies in bodywork. In 1998 she obtained a degree from the New Hampshire Institute for Therapeutic Arts, School of Massage Therapy. She has extensive training in bodywork with certification in cranial sacral techniques, lymphatic drainage, reflexology, and LaStone Therapy, to name a few.

While at Palmer College, Dr. Clark worked in the biochemistry department. Her love for cellular function has grown over the years. When she graduated from Palmer college in 2004, she opened a practice in Andalusia, Illinois. She noticed that not all chiropractic patients were getting well. She started putting together the missing pieces of regaining health at that time. She sold the practice in 2009, prior to moving back to her New Hampshire roots.

In 2010, Dr. Clark graduated from the Boston School of Herbal Studies and started Back to Life, LLC, which provides chiropractic care, reiki, massage therapy, and health coaching to patients in the local area. She has helped patients who have rare diseases or conditions that have been challenging for other practitioners to figure out. She attributes it to her love of biochemistry. Practicing in multiple health fields has contributed to her growing success.

To find out more, please visit:

www.backtolifenh.com

Made in USA - North Chelmsford, MA
647743_9780988447165
09.13.2022 1222